GLUCOSE REVOLUTION DIET COOKBOOK 2024

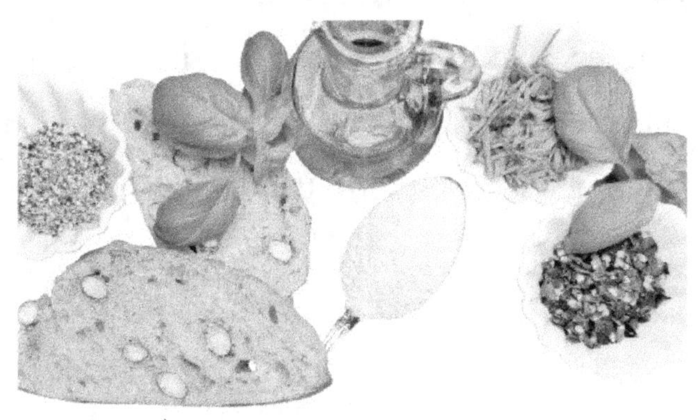

Discover Delicious Recipes for a Healthier Lifestyle

MISTY J. FONT

TABLE OF CONTENT

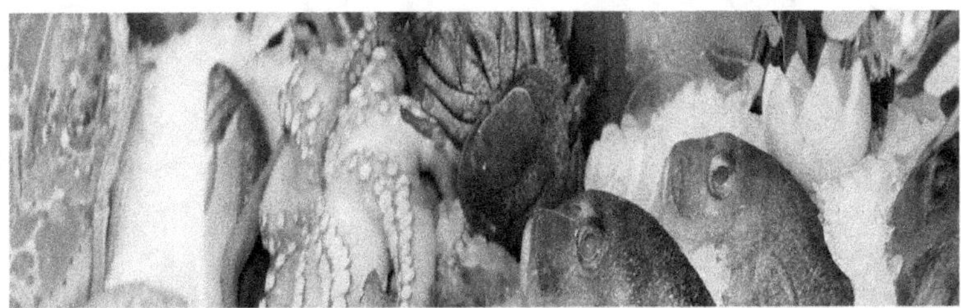

INTRODUCTION

In the curious town of Willow Brook, settled between moving slopes and a quiet stream, lived Jeremy, a man determined to recover his wellbeing and imperativeness. Jeremy's process started when he got a conclusion that would steer his life — an acknowledgment that his blood glucose levels were straying into concerning an area. Confronted with the possibility of a wellbeing challenge, Jeremy set out on a mission for an answer that wouldn't just deal with his glucose levels yet additionally change his relationship with food.

It was during a standard visit to the neighborhood book shop that Jeremy's eyes got the energetic front of the Glucose Insurgency Diet Cookbook. Interested by the commitment of a culinary experience that could line up with his wellbeing objectives, he chose to dig into its pages and investigate the potential outcomes inside.

As Jeremy flipped through the cookbook, he was welcomed by an ensemble of captivating recipes and an abundance of information about the Glucose Upheaval — a methodology that underlined the effect of nourishment on blood glucose levels. The opening chapters addressed Jeremy's concerns directly by dispelling myths, providing information on the science behind blood glucose management, and laying the groundwork for a diet that is both healthy and enjoyable.

Persuaded by a craving to assume command over his wellbeing, Jeremy focused on submerging himself in the Glucose Transformation Diet Cookbook. He moved toward the excursion not as a prohibitive eating routine but rather as a culinary investigation, anxious to find the rich embroidery of flavors that could coincide with his wellbeing goals.

Part by section, Jeremy explored through the cookbook's carefully arranged content. He figured out how to stock his kitchen with fundamentals that lined up with the Glucose Transformation way of life, changing his storage space into a sanctuary of supporting fixings. Brilliant shopping tips and a manual for deciphering names turned into his partners as he wandered into nearby business sectors, pursuing informed decisions that resounded with the standards of the Glucose Upheaval.

The recipes in the book were the heart of the book. Each one is a masterpiece that has been carefully crafted with balanced nutrition and exquisite taste in mind. For Jeremy, morning meals turned into a festival of empowering choices, with high-fiber and protein-pressed dinners establishing the vibe for his day. The fragrance of healthy snacks drifted through his kitchen, making a noontime desert garden of supplement thick guilty pleasure. Feeding suppers, one-pot ponders that moved on his taste buds, turned into the foundation of night feasts imparted to loved ones.

However, the Glucose Transformation was not only about feasts; it was a comprehensive way of life change. Jeremy embraced the recommendations for physical activity, incorporating fitness routines into his day and understanding the synergy between movement and glucose management. The cookbook's direction on exploring feasting out and overseeing get-togethers became priceless apparatuses, engaging Jeremy to settle on savvy decisions without settling on the delight of shared dinners.

As weeks transformed into months, Jeremy's devotion proved to be fruitful. His normal check-ups uncovered a perceptible improvement in his blood glucose levels, a demonstration of the groundbreaking force of the Glucose Transformation way of life. Past the numbers, Jeremy felt a recently discovered imperativeness flowing through his veins — an essentialness energized by deliberate nourishment, careful development, and a cheerful association with food.

Jeremy's story isn't simply a demonstration of the Glucose Unrest Diet Cookbook however to the flexibility of the human soul when filled by information, assurance, and the creativity of healthy living. In the peaceful town of Willow Creek, surrounded by rolling hills and the gentle gurgling of the river, Jeremy's journey serves as a source of inspiration and a beacon of hope for people who want more than just recovery—they want a life full of life and meaning.

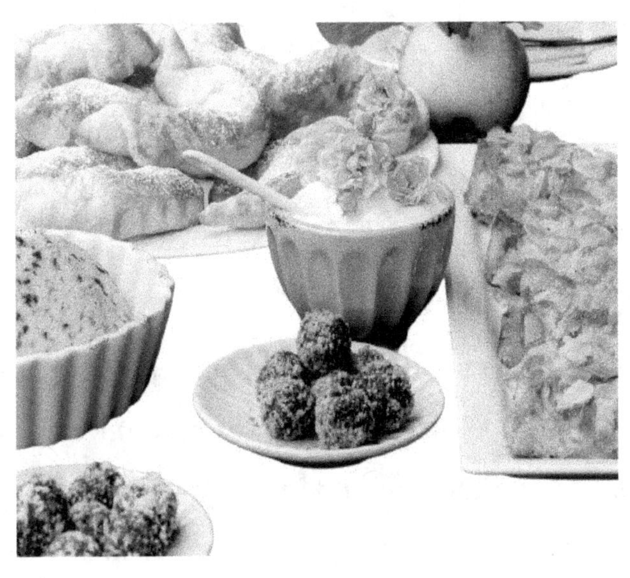

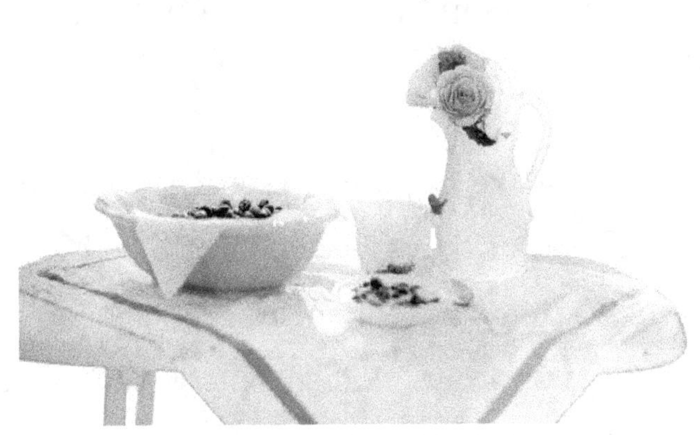

CHAPTER 1: UNDERSTANDING THE GLUCOSE REVOLUTION

Welcome to the basic part of our culinary campaign into the Glucose Transformation, where we disentangle the complexities of blood glucose levels and leave on an excursion towards ideal wellbeing and essentialness.

The Science Behind Blood Glucose Levels

At the core of the Glucose Upset lies a significant comprehension of the science behind blood glucose levels. Dive into the entrancing components that administer how our bodies interaction sugars, opening the insider facts that interface our dietary decisions to the rhythmic movement of energy flowing through our veins. By demystifying the science, we engage ourselves to pursue informed choices that resound with our special physiological requirements.

Exploring the Impact of Different Foods on Blood Sugar

Go along with us on a gastronomic investigation as we explore the maze of food sources and their unmistakable consequences for glucose. Find the nuanced dance between starches, fats, and proteins, and how they impact the sensitive equilibrium of glucose in our circulatory system. From the quick flood of energy from specific food varieties to the supported delivery given by others, this part reveals the specialty of making feasts that blend with the rhythms of our bodies.

Benefits of Maintaining Stable Glucose Levels

Maintaining stable glucose levels emerges as a key protagonist in this narrative. Stability is the foundation of optimal health. Figure out how adjusted glucose levels add to supported energy, mental lucidity, and by and large prosperity. This involves more than just avoiding peaks and crashes; it's tied in with cultivating a climate where your body works at its ideal, permitting you to flourish in each part of life.

Debunking Common Myths About Glucose and Diet

It is essential to distinguish fact from fiction in a world saturated with nutritional advice. In this segment, we expose normal legends encompassing glucose and diet, giving lucidity on misguided judgments that might have ruined your excursion to a better way of life. From demystifying the idea of "good" and "terrible" sugars to scattering the thought that smart dieting approaches penance, we furnish you with information that enables your decisions.

As we dive into the complexities of the Glucose Upheaval, let this section act as the compass directing you through the unfamiliar domains of your dietary scene. Together, we embrace the information that fills our change — an excursion towards a daily existence where equilibrium, essentialness, and joy interweave consistently. Welcome to the domain of grasping, the foundation of the Glucose Upheaval.

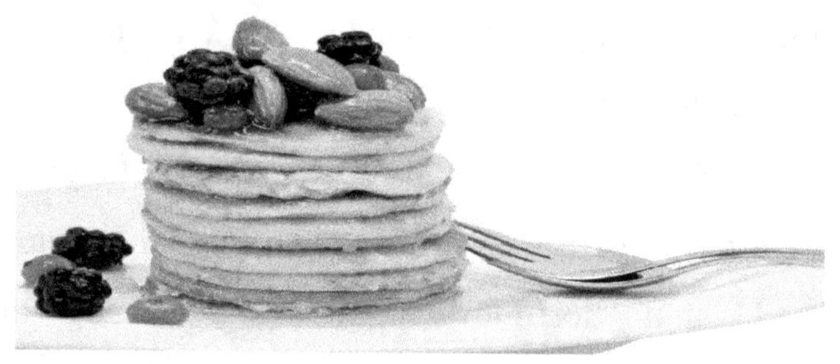

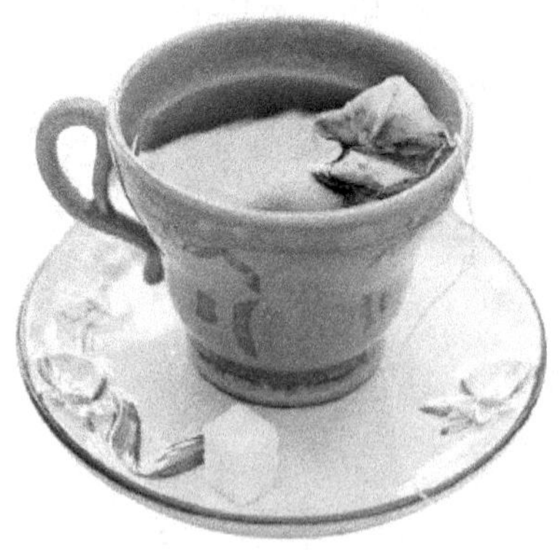

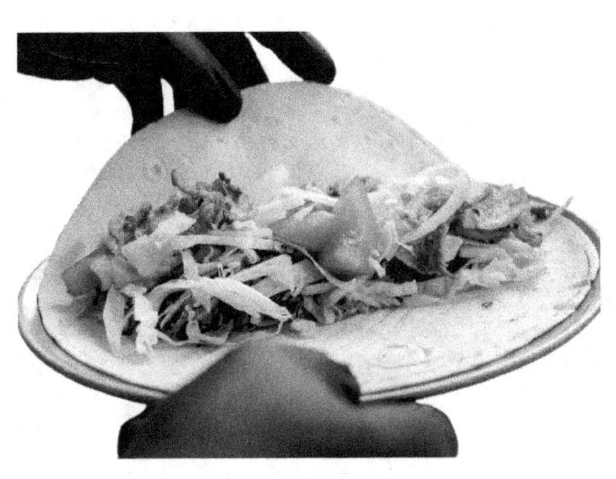

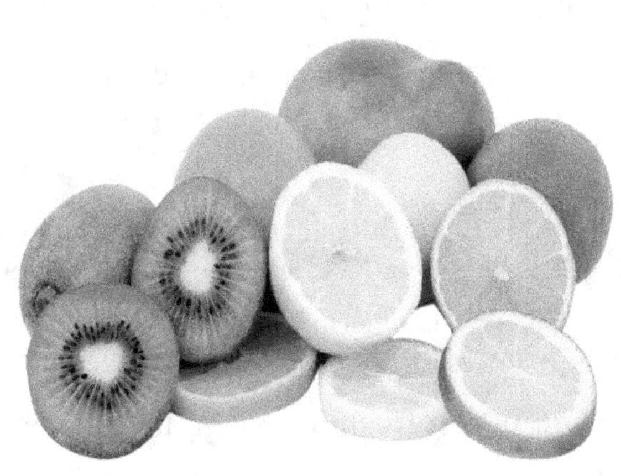

CHAPTER 2: THE GLUCOSE-FRIENDLY PANTRY

Welcome to the core of your culinary sanctuary — the Glucose-Accommodating Storeroom. In this section, we dig into the specialty of loading your kitchen for food as well as for progress on your Glucose Upheaval venture. We should investigate the fundamental structure hinders that will enable you to make feeding and delightful feasts, while holding your glucose levels under control.

Stocking Your Kitchen for Success

An exceptional kitchen is the material whereupon we create our refreshing magnum opuses. Come along with us as we walk you through the essential components of a successful pantry. Learn how to select the components of a Glucose Revolution diet, including whole grains, lean proteins, and a variety of colorful, nutrient-dense vegetables.

Essential Pantry Staples for a Glucose Revolution Lifestyle

Discover the treasures that adorn a Glucose-Friendly Pantry's shelves. Find the flexible universe of healthy grains, the protein-stuffed potential outcomes of vegetables, and the abundance of spices and flavors that raise flavor without settling for less on wellbeing. With our cautiously arranged rundown of fundamental staples, you'll have the apparatuses to make dinners that entice your taste buds as well as support your body from the inside.

Smart Shopping Tips and Label Reading Guide

Leave on your next supermarket experience outfitted with information. We'll furnish you with shrewd shopping tips to explore the paths, assisting you with pursuing informed choices that line up with your Glucose Unrest objectives. Interpret food marks with our far reaching guide, engaging you to pick items that help stable glucose levels without forfeiting flavor or assortment.

Meal Planning Strategies for Blood Sugar Control

The foundation of a fruitful Glucose Unrest lies in smart dinner arranging. Figure out how to make adjusted and fulfilling feasts that hold your glucose levels under wraps. From careful distributing to integrating an assortment of nutrition types into your everyday collection, our dinner arranging procedures offer you a guide to culinary achievement. Whether you're a carefully prepared feast prep fan or a fledgling in the kitchen, these procedures will smooth out your excursion towards better eating.

Imagine a place where each ingredient is a building block for a healthier you as we open the doors to your Glucose-Friendly Pantry. Allow this part to be your manual for changing your kitchen into a center of sustenance, imagination, and prosperity. Welcome to a reality where your storeroom turns into a strong partner on your Glucose Insurgency experience.

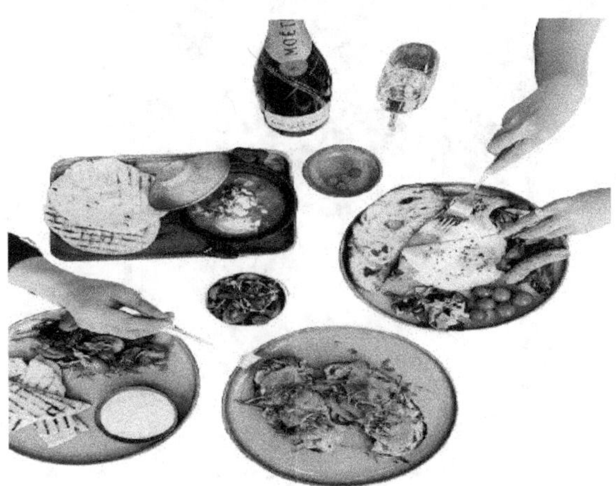

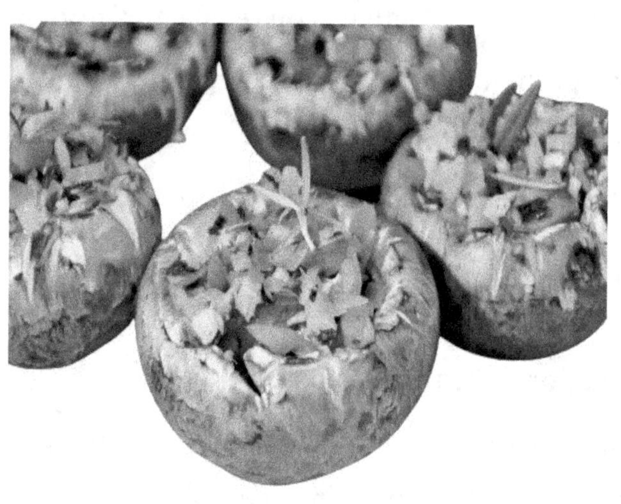

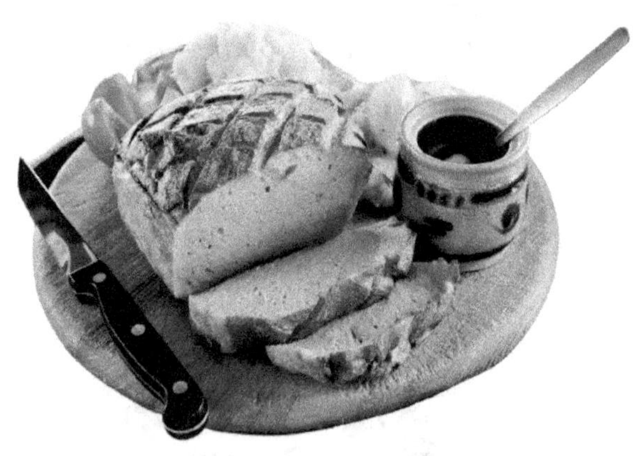

CHAPTER 3: ENERGIZING BREAKFASTS

Quinoa Berry Breakfast Bowl

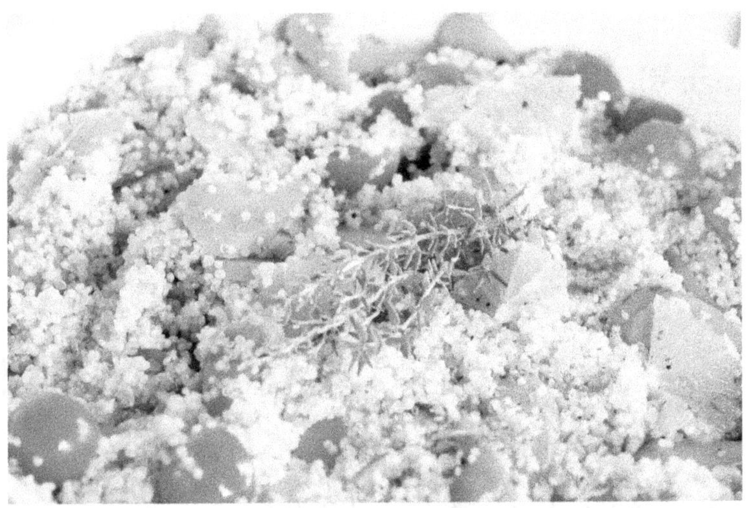

Description:

Raise your morning with this supplement pressed breakfast bowl highlighting quinoa, new berries, and a sprinkle of honey. It's a heavenly mix of surfaces and flavors, giving an eruption of energy to launch your day.

Serving Size: 1

Prep Time: 5 minutes

Cooking Time: 15 minutes

Ingredients:

- 1/2 cup quinoa
- 1 cup almond milk
- 1 cup mixed berries (strawberries, blueberries, raspberries)
- 1 tablespoon honey
- 1 tablespoon chia seeds
- A handful of sliced almonds

Instructions:

1. Wash quinoa and cook as indicated by bundle directions with almond milk.
2. Once cooked, move to a bowl and top with blended berries, chia seeds, cut almonds, and a sprinkle of honey.

3. Delicately blend and partake in your empowering breakfast!

Avocado & Egg Breakfast Wrap

Description:

Fuel your morning with this protein-pressed breakfast wrap. Velvety avocado, fried eggs, and a dash of salsa make a fantastic and nutritious dinner that is ideal for those in a hurry mornings.

Serving Size: 1

Prep Time: 10 minutes

Cooking Time: 5 minutes

Ingredients:

- 1 whole-grain wrap
- 1 ripe avocado, sliced
- 2 eggs, scrambled
- 1/4 cup salsa
- Salt and pepper to taste
- Fresh cilantro for garnish (optional)

Instructions:

1. Scramble eggs in a skillet with a touch of salt and pepper.
2. Spread out the entire grain wrap and layer with cut avocado and fried eggs.
3. Wrap it up, garnish with salsa and fresh cilantro, and enjoy!

Greek Yogurt Parfait with Granola

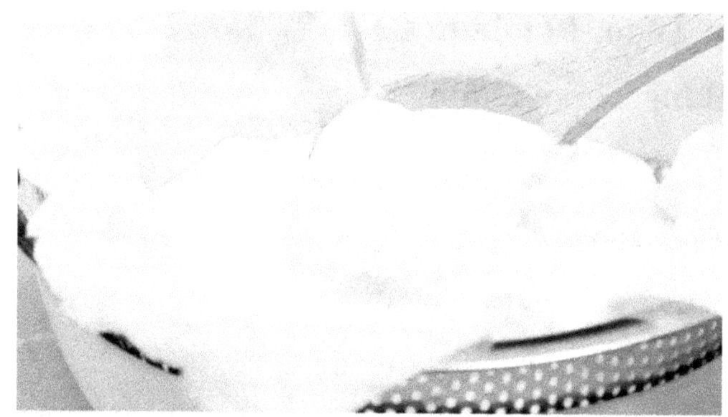

Description:

Enjoy a parfait that weds the smoothness of Greek yogurt with the mash of granola. Layered with new organic product, a great blend of surfaces and flavors fulfills your taste buds and gives a protein support.

Serving Size: 1

Prep Time: 5 minutes

Cooking Time: 0 minutes

Ingredients:

- 1 cup Greek yogurt
- 1/2 cup granola
- 1/2 cup mixed berries (strawberries, blueberries)
- 1 tablespoon honey
- A sprinkle of chia seeds

Instructions:

1. In a glass or bowl, layer Greek yogurt, granola, and blended berries.
2. Sprinkle with chia seeds and drizzle with honey.
3. Rehash layers and top with extra berries.

Sweet Potato and Spinach Breakfast Hash

Description:

This savory breakfast hash of poached eggs, sweet potatoes, and spinach will give you a boost in the morning. Loaded with fiber and supplements, a good choice keeps you full and centered.

Serving Size: 2

Prep Time: 10 minutes

Cooking Time: 20 minutes

Ingredients:

- 2 medium sweet potatoes, diced
- 2 cups fresh spinach
- 4 eggs
- 1 tablespoon olive oil
- Salt and pepper to taste

- Paprika for garnish

Instructions:

1. In a skillet, heat olive oil and sauté yams until brilliant brown and cooked through.

2. Add new spinach and cook until shriveled.

3. Crack eggs into wells that are made in the mixture. Cover and cook until eggs are finished.

4. Sprinkle paprika on top and season with salt and pepper. Serve and enjoy the flavors!

Banana Nut Overnight Oats

Description:

Get ready for a bustling morning by preparing these brilliant banana nut for the time being oats the prior night. The oats ingest the flavors for the time being, making a delightful and empowering breakfast.

Serving Size: 1

Prep Time: 5 minutes (plus overnight soaking)

Cooking Time: 0 minutes

Ingredients:

- 1/2 cup rolled oats
- 1/2 cup almond milk
- 1 ripe banana, mashed
- 2 tablespoons chopped nuts (walnuts, almonds)
- 1 tablespoon honey
- A dash of cinnamon

Instructions:

1. In a container, join moved oats, almond milk, crushed banana, cleaved nuts, honey, and cinnamon.
2. Cover and refrigerate overnight, stirring well.
3. Toward the beginning of the day, give it a decent mix and partake in your easy and nutritious breakfast!

Spinach and Feta Breakfast Wrap

Description:

Start off your day with an exquisite spinach and feta breakfast wrap. It's a quick and filling option for those busy mornings, packed with vitamins and protein.

Serving Size: 1

Prep Time: 10 minutes

Cooking Time: 5 minutes

Ingredients:

- 1 whole-grain wrap
- 2 eggs, scrambled
- 1 cup fresh spinach
- 1/4 cup crumbled feta cheese
- Salt and pepper to taste
- Salsa for garnish (optional)

Instructions:

1. Scramble eggs in a container with a spot of salt and pepper.

2. Spread out the entire grain wrap and layer with new spinach and fried eggs.

3. Sprinkle with disintegrated feta and add salsa whenever wanted. Enjoy your protein-rich breakfast by rolling it up!

Chia Seed Pudding with Berries

Description:

Enjoy a rich and nutritious chia seed pudding finished off with lively berries. This morning meal isn't just a dining experience for the eyes yet in addition a rich wellspring of omega-3 unsaturated fats and cell reinforcements.

Serving Size: 2

Prep Time: 5 minutes (plus chilling time)

Cooking Time: 0 minutes

Ingredients:

- 1/2 cup chia seeds

- 2 cups almond milk

- 1 teaspoon vanilla extract

- 2 tablespoons maple syrup

- 1 cup mixed berries (blueberries, raspberries)

Instructions:

1. In a bowl, whisk together chia seeds, almond milk, vanilla concentrate, and maple syrup.

2. Refrigerate for no less than 2 hours or short-term until it arrives at a pudding-like consistency.

3. Serve in bowls with mixed berries on top. Partake in this nutritious and fulfilling pudding!

Egg and Veggie Breakfast Muffins

Description:

These egg and veggie breakfast biscuits are the exemplification of comfort and sustenance. Loaded with protein and a grouping of brilliant vegetables, they're ideally suited for an in and out morning.

Serving Size: 4 muffins

Prep Time: 10 minutes

Cooking Time: 20 minutes

Ingredients:

- 6 eggs, beaten
- 1/2 cup bell peppers, diced (assorted colors)
- 1/2 cup cherry tomatoes, halved
- 1/4 cup red onion, finely chopped
- 1/4 cup feta cheese, crumbled
- Salt and pepper to taste
- Fresh parsley for garnish

Instructions:

1. Preheat the stove to 350°F (175°C) and oil a biscuit tin.

2. Beat eggs, add diced bell peppers, cherry tomatoes, red onion, and crumbled feta to a bowl. Add salt and pepper to taste.

3. Empty the combination into the biscuit tin and heat for 20 minutes or until the eggs are set.

4. Decorate with new parsley and partake in these wonderful breakfast biscuits!

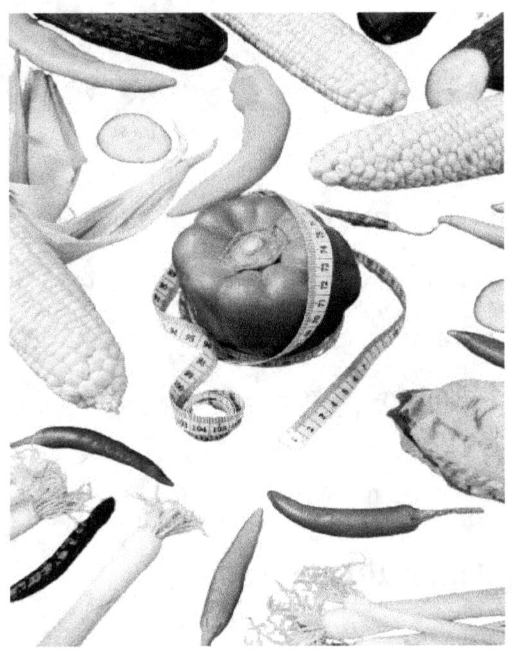

Cinnamon Apple Quinoa Porridge

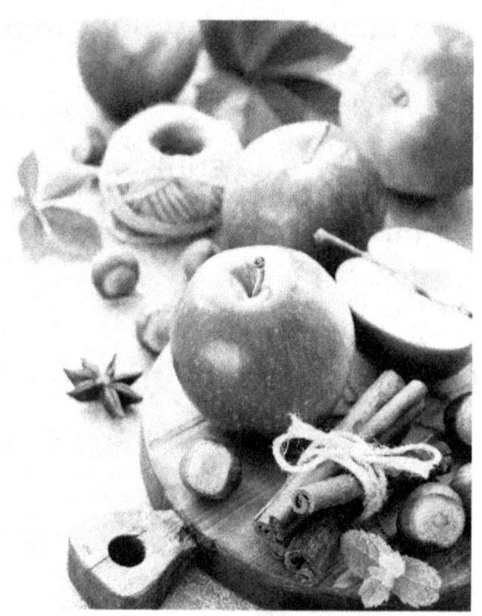

Description:

Warm up your morning with a consoling bowl of cinnamon apple quinoa porridge. This good and tasty choice is a great curve on conventional cereal, offering a protein-pressed start to your day.

Serving Size: 2

Prep Time: 5 minutes

Cooking Time: 20 minutes

Ingredients:

- 1/2 cup quinoa

- 1 cup almond milk

- 1 apple, diced

- 1 tablespoon maple syrup

- 1/2 teaspoon cinnamon

- A pinch of nutmeg

- Chopped walnuts for garnish

Instructions:

1. Wash quinoa and cook as per bundle guidelines with almond milk.

2. In a different container, sauté diced apples with maple syrup, cinnamon, and nutmeg until delicate.

3. In a bowl, combine the apple mixture with the cooked quinoa.

4. Decorate with cleaved pecans and a sprinkle of maple syrup. Partake in this comfortable and nutritious porridge!

Blueberry Almond Chia Pudding

Description:

Enjoy the decency of blueberries and almonds in this scrumptious chia pudding. Wealthy in cell reinforcements and omega-3 unsaturated fats, it's a great and nutritious breakfast choice.

Serving Size: 2

Prep Time: 5 minutes (plus chilling time)

Cooking Time: 0 minutes

Ingredients:

- 1/2 cup chia seeds
- 2 cups almond milk
- 1 teaspoon almond extract
- 2 tablespoons honey
- 1 cup blueberries (fresh or frozen)
- Sliced almonds for garnish

Instructions:

1. In a bowl, whisk together chia seeds, almond milk, almond concentrate, and honey.

2. Refrigerate for no less than 2 hours or short-term until it arrives at a pudding-like consistency.

3. Layer the chia pudding with blueberries in serving glasses.

4. Embellish with cut almonds and partake in this cell reinforcement rich and fulfilling pudding

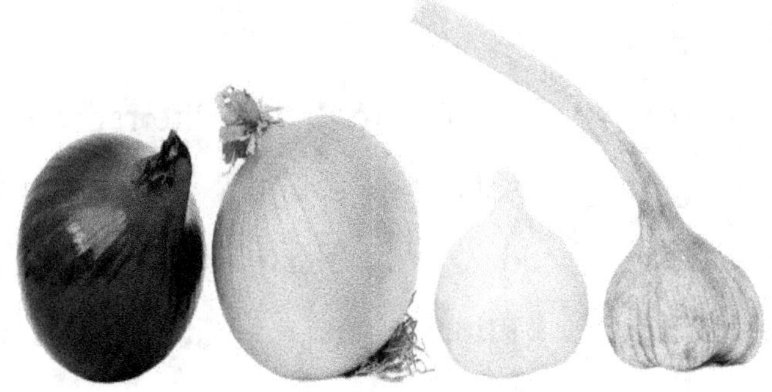

Chapter 4: Wholesome Lunches

Mediterranean Quinoa Salad Bowl

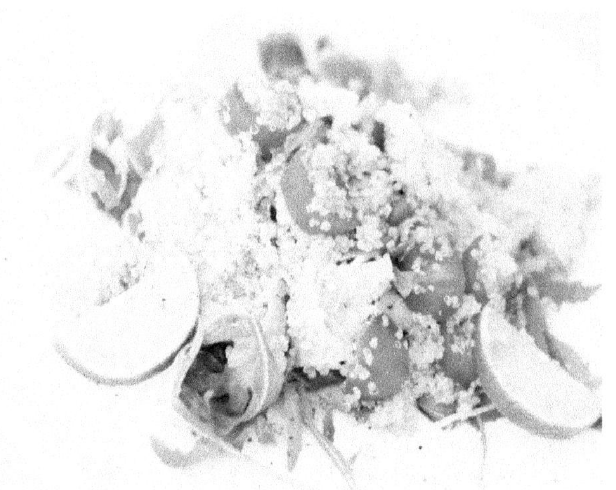

Description:

Transport your taste buds to the Mediterranean with this lively quinoa salad bowl. Loaded with beautiful veggies, feta cheddar, and a fiery lemon vinaigrette, a healthy and fulfilling lunch gives an explosion of flavors.

Serving Size: 2

Prep Time: 15 minutes

Cooking Time: 20 minutes

Ingredients:

- 1 cup quinoa
- 2 cups cherry tomatoes, halved
- 1 cucumber, diced
- 1/2 cup Kalamata olives, sliced
- 1/2 cup feta cheese, crumbled
- 1/4 cup red onion, finely chopped
- Fresh parsley for garnish

For the dressing:

- 3 tablespoons olive oil,
- 2 tablespoons lemon juice, salt,
- and pepper to taste

Instructions:

1. Cook quinoa as per bundle guidelines and let it cool.
2. In an enormous bowl, join quinoa, cherry tomatoes, cucumber, olives, feta cheddar, and red onion.

3. Pour the dressing over the salad and whisk it together. Throw tenderly.

4. Embellish with new parsley and partake in this supplement thick Mediterranean joy!

Grilled Chicken and Vegetable Wrap

Description:

Relish the effortlessness of a barbecued chicken and vegetable wrap. This lunch choice consolidates lean protein with different vivid veggies, making a flavorful and adjusted feast that fulfills your late morning desires.

Serving Size: 1

Prep Time: 10 minutes

Cooking Time: 15 minutes

Ingredients:

- 1 boneless, skinless chicken breast
- 1 whole-grain wrap

- 1/2 cup bell peppers, sliced (assorted colors)
- 1/2 cup zucchini, thinly sliced
- 1 tablespoon olive oil
- Salt and pepper to taste
- Hummus for spreading

Instructions:

1. Use salt and pepper to season the chicken breast.
2. Barbecue the chicken until cooked through, around 7-8 minutes for every side.
3. In a different skillet, sauté chime peppers and zucchini in olive oil until delicate.
4. Spread hummus overall grain wrap, add cut barbecued chicken, and top with sautéed vegetables. Roll up and partake in this healthy wrap!

Salmon and Quinoa Stuffed Bell Peppers

Description:

Raise your lunch with these bright and supplement pressed salmon and quinoa stuffed chime peppers. Overflowing with Omega-3 unsaturated fats and protein, a balanced dinner leaves you feeling fulfilled and sustained.

Serving Size: 4

Prep Time: 20 minutes

Cooking Time: 30 minutes

Ingredients:

- 1 cup quinoa
- 4 bell peppers, halved and seeds removed
- 1 pound salmon fillet, cooked and flaked
- 1 cup cherry tomatoes, diced
- 1/2 cup feta cheese, crumbled
- Fresh dill for garnish

For the dressing:

- 3 tablespoons olive oil,
- 2 tablespoons balsamic vinegar,
- salt, and pepper to taste

Instructions:

1. Cook quinoa as per bundle guidelines.
2. In a bowl, blend quinoa, chipped salmon, cherry tomatoes, and feta cheddar.
3. Divide the mixture among the bell pepper halves.
4. Whisk together the dressing fixings and sprinkle over the stuffed peppers.
5. Heat in a preheated broiler at 375°F (190°C) for 25-30 minutes or until peppers are delicate.
6. Decorate with new dill and relish this healthy and delightful lunch!

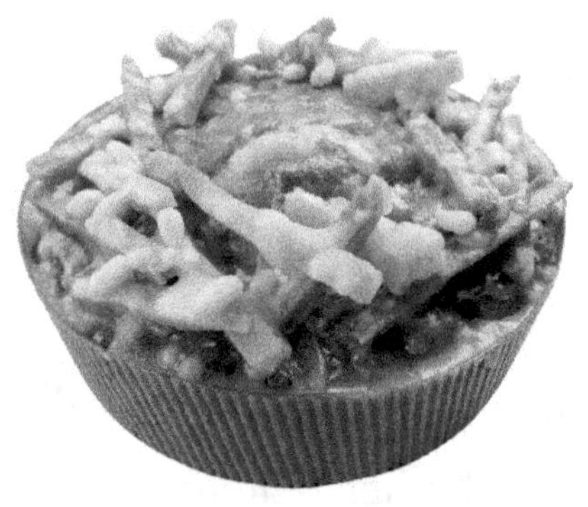

Chickpea and Vegetable Stir-Fry

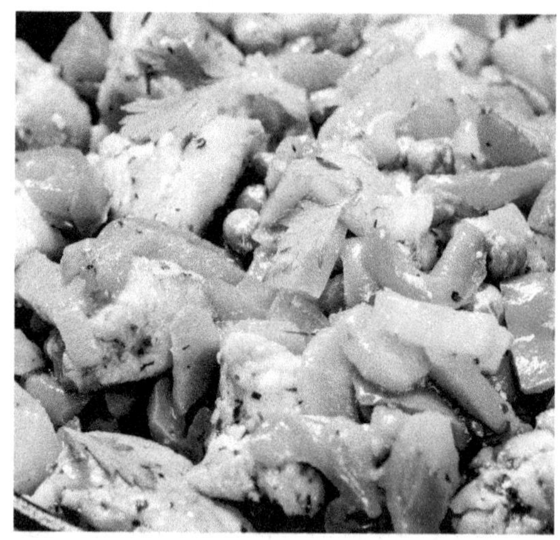

Description:

Set out on a culinary excursion with this lively chickpea and vegetable sautéed food. Loaded with protein and a variety of brilliant veggies, it's a speedy and nutritious choice for a late morning feast.

Serving Size: 2

Prep Time: 15 minutes

Cooking Time: 15 minutes

Ingredients:

- 1 can chickpeas, drained and rinsed
- 2 cups broccoli florets
- 1 red bell pepper, sliced
- 1 carrot, julienned
- 2 tablespoons soy sauce
- 1 tablespoon sesame oil
- 1 tablespoon rice vinegar
- 1 teaspoon ginger, minced
- 2 cloves garlic, minced
- Sesame seeds for garnish

Instructions:

1. In a wok or huge dish, heat sesame oil and sauté ginger and garlic until fragrant.
2. Add broccoli, chime pepper, and carrot, sautéing until vegetables are delicate fresh.
3. Mix in chickpeas, soy sauce, and rice vinegar. Cook until warmed through.
4. Decorate with sesame seeds and relish this vivid and supplement thick pan fried food!

Caprese Quinoa Bowl

Description:

Experience the exemplary Caprese salad in a generous quinoa bowl. With the expansion of quinoa, this lunch turns into a healthy, protein-pressed dish that is both fulfilling and brimming with new flavors.

Serving Size: 2

Prep Time: 10 minutes

Cooking Time: 15 minutes

Ingredients:

- 1 cup quinoa
- 1 cup cherry tomatoes, halved
- 1 cup fresh mozzarella balls, halved
- 1/4 cup fresh basil, chopped
- 2 tablespoons balsamic glaze
- Salt and pepper to taste
- Extra virgin olive oil for drizzling

Instructions:

1. Cook quinoa as indicated by bundle guidelines.
2. Mix cooked quinoa, cherry tomatoes, mozzarella, and chopped basil in a bowl.
3. Sprinkle with balsamic coating, olive oil, and season with salt and pepper.
4. Throw delicately and partake in this light yet filling Caprese quinoa bowl!

Turkey and Avocado Lettuce Wraps

Description:

For a low-carb, high-flavor lunch, enjoy these turkey and avocado lettuce wraps. They are a refreshing and well-balanced choice for lunch because they are loaded with healthy fats and lean protein.

Serving Size: 2

Prep Time: 10 minutes

Cooking Time: 0 minutes

Ingredients:

- 1/2 pound turkey breast, sliced
- 1 avocado, sliced
- 1 cup cherry tomatoes, diced
- 1/4 cup red onion, finely chopped
- 2 tablespoons Greek yogurt
- Fresh cilantro for garnish
- Large lettuce leaves for wrapping

Instructions:

1. Spread out the lettuce leaves and equitably disseminate turkey cuts on each.

2. Sliced avocado, red onion, cherry tomatoes, and Greek yogurt on top.

3. Embellish with new cilantro and fold the lettuce over the filling. Partake in these light and tasty turkey and avocado wraps!

Sweet Potato and Chickpea Buddha Bowl

Description:

Support your body with a vivid and supplement rich yam and chickpea Buddha bowl. Loaded with plant-based protein and different veggies, it's a delightful and outwardly engaging lunch choice.

Serving Size: 2

Prep Time: 15 minutes

Cooking Time: 25 minutes

Ingredients:

- 2 sweet potatoes, diced
- 1 can chickpeas, drained and rinsed
- 1 cup broccoli florets
- 1/2 red onion, sliced
- 2 tablespoons olive oil
- 1 teaspoon cumin
- 1/2 teaspoon paprika
- Salt and pepper to taste
- Tahini sauce for drizzling

Instructions:

1. Throw yams, chickpeas, broccoli, and red onion with olive oil, cumin, paprika, salt, and pepper.
2. Bake at 400 degrees Fahrenheit (200 degrees Celsius) for 25 minutes, or until golden and crispy.

3. Partition the broiled fixings into bowls and sprinkle with tahini sauce. Take pleasure in this tasty and nutritious Buddha bowl!

Lentil and Vegetable Soup

Description:

In the afternoon, warm up with a hearty lentil and vegetable soup. Stacked with fiber, protein, and various veggies, it's a relieving and supplement thick decision for a sound lunch.

Serving Size: 4

Prep Time: 15 minutes

Cooking Time: 30 minutes

Ingredients:

- 1 cup dry lentils, rinsed
- 1 onion, diced
- 2 carrots, sliced
- 2 celery stalks, chopped

- 3 cloves garlic, minced
- 1 can diced tomatoes
- 6 cups vegetable broth
- 1 teaspoon cumin
- 1/2 teaspoon thyme
- Salt and pepper to taste
- Fresh parsley for garnish

Instructions:

1. In a huge pot, sauté onions, carrots, and celery until mellowed.
2. Add garlic, lentils, diced tomatoes, vegetable stock, cumin, thyme, salt, and pepper.
3. Reduce the heat and simmer for 25 to 30 minutes, or until the lentils are tender.
4. Decorate with new parsley and enjoy this healthy and supporting lentil and vegetable soup!

Shrimp and Quinoa Salad

Description:

Hoist your noon experience with a reviving shrimp and quinoa salad. Loaded with protein, vegetables, and a fiery dressing, it's a light yet fulfilling choice for a reasonable late morning feast.

Serving Size: 2

Prep Time: 20 minutes

Cooking Time: 15 minutes

Ingredients:

- 1 cup quinoa
- 1/2 pound shrimp, peeled and deveined
- 1 cup cherry tomatoes, halved
- 1 cucumber, diced
- 1/4 cup red onion, finely chopped
- 1/4 cup feta cheese, crumbled
- Fresh mint for garnish

For the dressing:

- 3 tablespoons olive oil,
- 2 tablespoons lemon juice,

- 1 teaspoon Dijon mustard, salt, and pepper to taste

Instructions:

- Cook quinoa as per bundle guidelines and let it cool.

- Season shrimp with salt and pepper and sauté until cooked through.

- Combine the quinoa, shrimp, cucumber, red onion, cherry tomatoes, and feta cheese in a large bowl.

- Whisk together the dressing fixings and pour over the serving of mixed greens. Gently toss.

- Enjoy this light and flavorful shrimp and quinoa salad by garnishing with fresh mint!

These healthy lunch recipes are created to furnish you with a brilliant mix of flavors, supplements, and fulfillment. May each nibble add to a decent and sustaining way of life as you keep on embracing the Glucose Unrest.

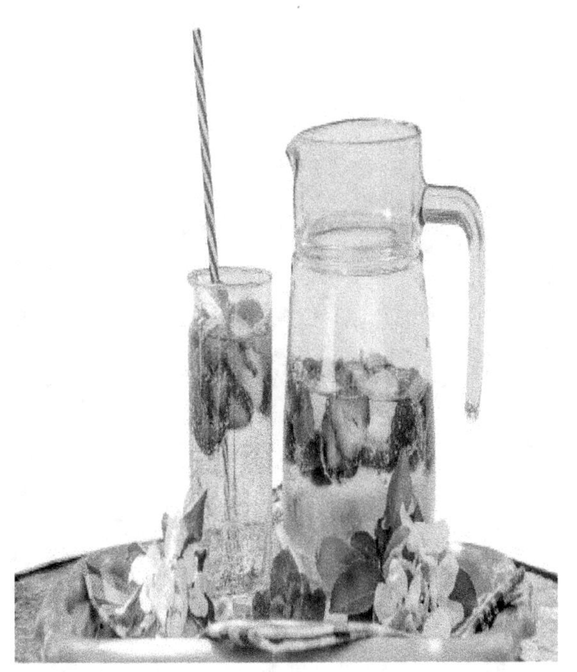

Chapter 5: Nourishing Dinners

Baked Lemon Herb Salmon

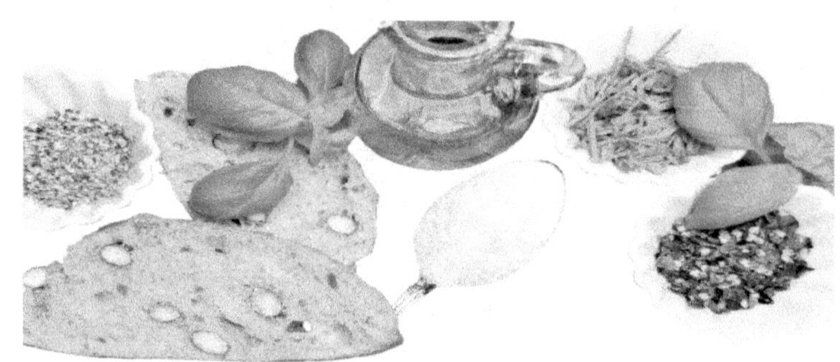

Description:

Enjoy the delicious kinds of heated lemon spice salmon, a supper choice that is both brilliant and supplement stuffed. This dish is a filling centerpiece for your evening meal because of its perfect harmony between zesty lemon and aromatic herbs.

Serving Size: 4

Prep Time: 10 minutes

Cooking Time: 20 minutes

Ingredients:

- 4 salmon fillets
- 2 tablespoons olive oil
- Zest and juice of 1 lemon
- 2 cloves garlic, minced
- 1 tablespoon fresh dill, chopped
- Salt and pepper to taste
- Lemon wedges for serving

Instructions:

1. Preheat the broiler to 400°F (200°C) and line a baking sheet with material paper.
2. Put salmon filets on the sheet and brush with olive oil.
3. Blend lemon zing, lemon juice, minced garlic, hacked dill, salt, and pepper.
4. Spoon the blend over the salmon.
5. Heat for 20 minutes or until the salmon is cooked through.

6. Present with lemon wedges and partake in this tasty supper!

Vegetarian Chickpea Curry

Description:

Enjoy the rich and sweet-smelling kinds of a vegan chickpea curry for a wonderful and plant-based supper. Overflowing with flavors and healthy fixings, this curry is both consoling and sustaining.

Serving Size: 4

Prep Time: 15 minutes

Cooking Time: 25 minutes

Ingredients:

- 2 cans chickpeas, drained and rinsed
- 1 onion, finely chopped
- 2 tomatoes, diced
- 1 cup coconut milk
- 2 tablespoons curry powder

- 1 teaspoon turmeric
- 1 teaspoon cumin
- 1 teaspoon coriander
- Salt and pepper to taste
- Fresh cilantro for garnish
- Cooked rice for serving

Instructions:

1. In a dish, sauté hacked onions until mellowed.
2. Add curry powder, turmeric, cumin, and coriander, mixing until fragrant.
3. Mix in diced tomatoes, chickpeas, and coconut milk.
4. Cook for twenty minutes.
5. Season with salt and pepper. Serve over cooked rice, decorated with new cilantro

Grilled Chicken and Quinoa Stuffed Bell Peppers

Description:

Raise your supper table with these barbecued chicken and quinoa stuffed chime peppers. Loaded with protein and fiber, this healthy dish is however outwardly engaging as it seems to be flavorful, making it an ideal choice for family meals.

Serving Size: 6

Prep Time: 20 minutes

Cooking Time: 30 minutes

Ingredients:

- 1 cup quinoa, cooked
- 1.5 pounds chicken breast, grilled and diced
- 6 bell peppers, halved and seeds removed
- 1 cup black beans, drained and rinsed
- 1 cup corn kernels
- 1 cup cherry tomatoes, diced

- 1 cup shredded cheddar cheese

- 1 teaspoon cumin

- 1 teaspoon chili powder

- Salt and pepper to taste

- Fresh cilantro for garnish

Instructions:

1. Preheat the broiler to 375°F (190°C) and oil a baking dish.

2. In a bowl, join quinoa, barbecued chicken, dark beans, corn, cherry tomatoes, destroyed cheddar, cumin, stew powder, salt, and pepper.

3. Stuff each chime pepper half with the blend and spot in the baking dish.

4. Prepare for 30 minutes or until the peppers are delicate.

5. Decorate with new cilantro and serve.

Spaghetti Squash Primavera

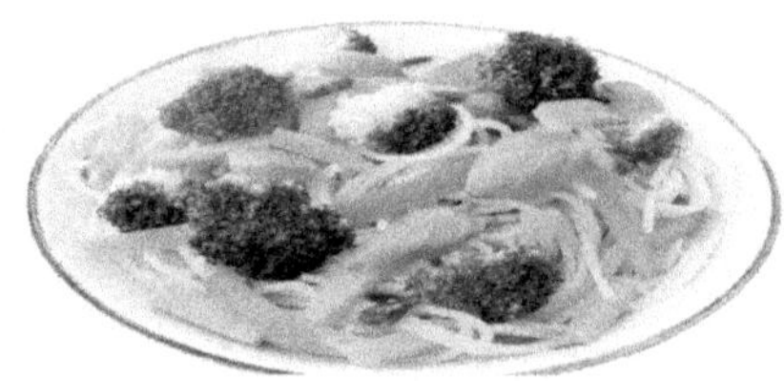

Description:

Experience the healthy integrity of spaghetti squash primavera, a low-carb option in contrast to conventional pasta dishes. Loaded with dynamic vegetables and exquisite flavors, this supper choice is a brilliant curve on a work of art.

Serving Size: 4

Prep Time: 15 minutes

Cooking Time: 40 minutes

Ingredients:

- 1 large spaghetti squash, halved and seeds removed
- 2 tablespoons olive oil
- 1 onion, thinly sliced

- 2 bell peppers, julienned (assorted colors)

- 2 zucchinis, julienned

- 1 cup cherry tomatoes, halved

- 3 cloves garlic, minced

- 1 teaspoon Italian seasoning

- Salt and pepper to taste

- Grated Parmesan cheese for garnish

- Fresh basil for garnish

Instructions:

1. Preheat the broiler to 400°F (200°C) and put spaghetti squash parts on a baking sheet.

2. Cook the squash for 30-40 minutes or until delicate.

3. In a container, sauté cut onions, julienned ringer peppers, zucchinis, and minced garlic in olive oil until mellowed.

4. Scratch the spaghetti squash into "noodles" and throw with sautéed vegetables.

5. Season with Italian flavoring, salt, and pepper.

6. Embellish with ground Parmesan cheddar and new basil.

7. Serve and partake in this feeding supper!

Teriyaki Tofu Stir-Fry

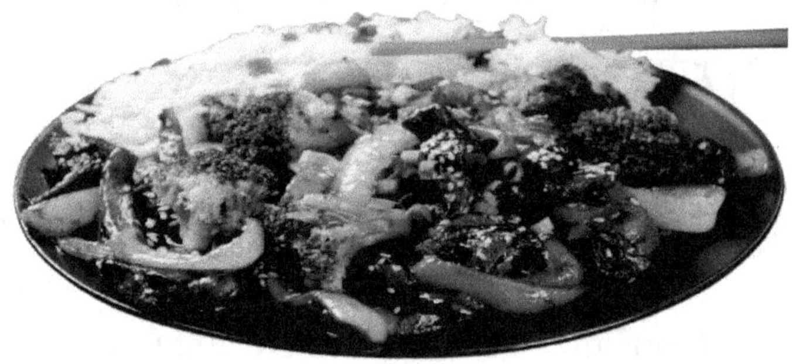

Description:

A protein-rich and flavorful teriyaki tofu stir-fry will delight your taste buds. Loaded with brilliant veggies and a flavorful sauce, this sautéed food is a delightful and healthy decision.

Serving Size: 3

Prep Time: 15 minutes

Cooking Time: 15 minutes

Ingredients:

- 1 block extra-firm tofu, pressed and cubed
- 1 cup broccoli florets
- 1 bell pepper, sliced (assorted colors)
- 1 carrot, julienned
- 1 cup snow peas, trimmed
- 2 tablespoons soy sauce
- 1 tablespoon hoisin sauce
- 1 tablespoon sesame oil
- 1 tablespoon rice vinegar
- 1 tablespoon honey
- 2 teaspoons cornstarch
- Sesame seeds for garnish
- Green onions for garnish

Instructions:

1. Cubed tofu should be sautéed until golden brown in a pan.

2. Include snow peas, carrot, broccoli, and bell pepper.

3. Pan sear until veggies are fresh delicate.

4. In a bowl, whisk together soy sauce, hoisin sauce, sesame oil, rice vinegar, honey, and cornstarch. Pour over the tofu and vegetables.

5. Throw until very much covered and sauce thickens.

6. Embellish with sesame seeds and green onions.

7. Serve over rice or noodles.

Healthy Chicken and Vegetable Sheet Pan Dinner

Description:

This healthy dinner on a sheet pan with chicken and vegetables will make dinner preparation easier. This one-pan wonder is loaded with vibrant vegetables and lean protein, provides a balanced and nourishing meal, and it makes cleanup simple.

Serving Size: 4

Prep Time: 15 minutes

Cooking Time: 25 minutes

Ingredients:

- 4 boneless, skinless chicken breasts
- 1 pound baby potatoes, halved
- 1 cup baby carrots
- 1 cup broccoli florets
- 1 cup cherry tomatoes, halved
- 2 tablespoons olive oil
- 1 teaspoon garlic powder
- 1 teaspoon onion powder
- 1 teaspoon dried thyme
- Salt and pepper to taste
- Fresh parsley for garnish

Instructions:

1. Prepare a baking sheet by lining it with parchment paper and preheating the oven to 425°F (220°C).

2. Place chicken bosoms, child potatoes, child carrots, broccoli, and cherry tomatoes on the sheet.

3. Sprinkle with salt, pepper, garlic powder, onion powder, dried thyme, and olive oil.

4. Throw to cover everything uniformly, then, at that point, spread into a solitary layer.

5. Heat for 25 minutes or until the chicken is cooked through. Serve while garnished with fresh parsley.

Stuffed Bell Peppers with Ground Turkey and Quinoa

Description:

Experience a generous and healthy supper with these stuffed chime peppers loaded up with a tasty combination of ground turkey and quinoa. This family-accommodating dish is both soothing and nutritious, making it an ideal expansion to your supper pivot.

Serving Size: 4

Prep Time: 20 minutes

Cooking Time: 40 minutes

Ingredients:

- 4 bell peppers, halved and seeds removed
- 1 cup quinoa, cooked
- 1 pound ground turkey
- 1 onion, finely chopped
- 2 cloves garlic, minced
- 1 can black beans, drained and rinsed
- 1 cup corn kernels
- 1 cup tomato sauce
- 1 teaspoon cumin

- 1 teaspoon chili powder

- Salt and pepper to taste

- Shredded cheddar cheese for topping

- Fresh cilantro for garnish

Instructions:

1. Preheat the broiler to 375°F (190°C) and oil a baking dish.

2. Cook the ground turkey, onions, and garlic in a pan until the meat is browned.

3. Add cooked quinoa, dark beans, corn, pureed tomatoes, cumin, stew powder, salt, and pepper.

4. Stew for 10 minutes.

5. The turkey and quinoa mixture should be put in each half of the bell pepper.

6. Top with destroyed cheddar and heat for 30 minutes or until peppers are delicate.

7. Decorate with new cilantro and serve.

Mushroom and Spinach Stuffed Chicken Breast

Description:

Raise your supper with these mushroom and spinach stuffed chicken bosoms. The blend of flavorful mushrooms, delicate spinach, and succulent chicken makes a delightful and outwardly engaging dish that is ideally suited for an extraordinary night feast.

Serving Size: 2

Prep Time: 15 minutes

Cooking Time: 30 minutes

Ingredients:

- 2 boneless, skinless chicken breasts
- 1 cup mushrooms, finely chopped
- 2 cups fresh spinach, chopped
- 1/2 cup feta cheese, crumbled
- 2 cloves garlic, minced

- 2 tablespoons olive oil

- Salt and pepper to taste

- Paprika for garnish

- Fresh parsley for garnish

Instructions:

1. Preheat the broiler to 375°F (190°C).

2. In a container, sauté mushrooms and garlic in olive oil until mellowed.

3. Add cleaved spinach and cook until shriveled.

4. Eliminate from intensity and mix in feta cheddar.

5. Cut a pocket into every chicken bosom and stuff with the mushroom and spinach combination.

6. The chicken breasts' exteriors should be seasoned with paprika, salt, and pepper.

7. Bake the chicken for 25 to 30 minutes, or until it is cooked through.

- Embellish with new parsley and serve.

Quinoa and Black Bean Stuffed Acorn Squash

Description:

Embrace the kinds of fall with these quinoa and dark bean stuffed oak seed squash. Loaded up with a nutritious combination of quinoa, dark beans, and pre-winter flavors, this supper choice is a good and fulfilling decision for a comfortable night dinner.

Serving Size: 4
Prep Time: 20 minutes
Cooking Time: 40 minutes

Ingredients:

- 2 acorn squash, halved and seeds removed
- 1 cup quinoa, cooked
- 1 can black beans, drained and rinsed

- 1/2 cup red onion, finely chopped
- 1/2 cup corn kernels
- 1 teaspoon cumin
- 1/2 teaspoon cinnamon
- Salt and pepper to taste
- 1/4 cup feta cheese, crumbled
- Fresh cilantro for garnish

Instructions:

1. Preheat the stove to 375°F (190°C) and line a baking sheet with material paper.
2. Bake the cut-side-down acorn squash halves for 20 minutes on the baking sheet.
3. In a bowl, blend cooked quinoa, dark beans, red onion, corn, cumin, cinnamon, salt, and pepper.
4. Flip the squash parts, stuff with the quinoa combination, and heat for 20 extra minutes.
5. Crush some feta cheese and sprinkle some fresh cilantro on top.

6. Serve this delicious and filling meal to your
    guests!

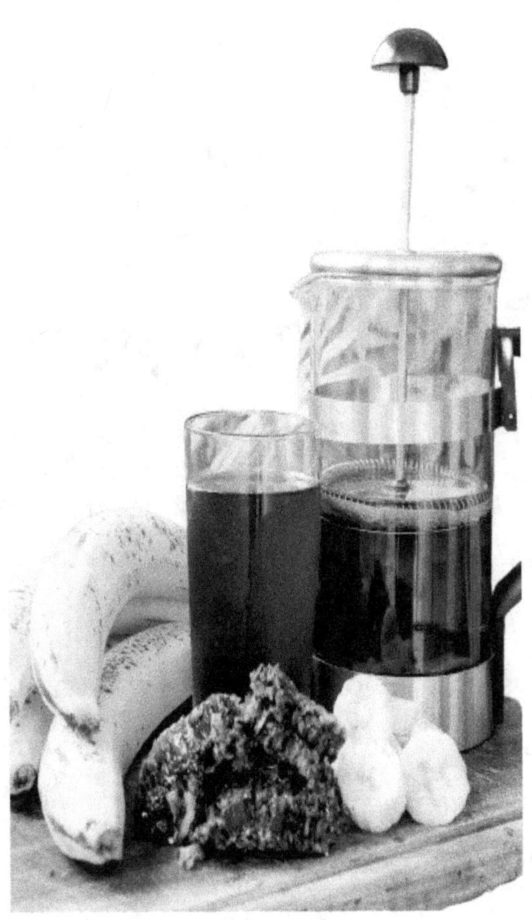

Chapter 6: Smart Snacking

Greek Yogurt Parfait with Berries

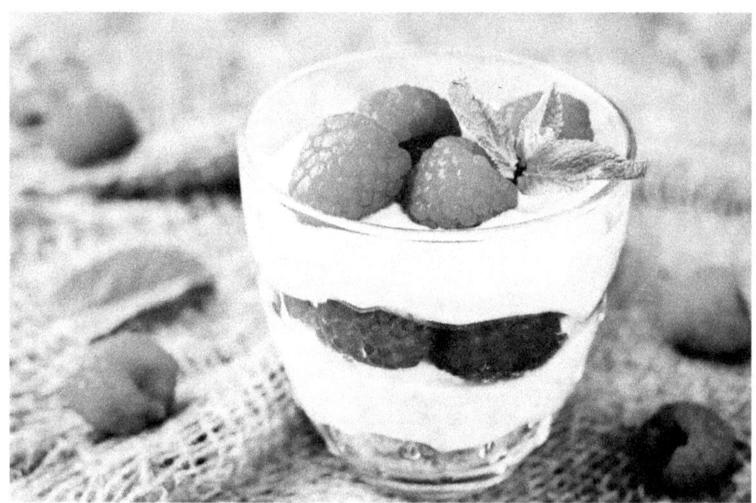

Description:

With this Greek Yogurt Parfait, you can indulge in a healthy snack option. Layered with smooth Greek yogurt, new berries, and a sprinkle of granola, this parfait is a great and nutritious treat to fulfill your sweet desires.

Serving Size: 1

Prep Time: 5 minutes

Cooking Time: 0 minutes

Ingredients:

- 1 cup Greek yogurt
- 1/2 cup mixed berries (strawberries, blueberries, raspberries)
- 2 tablespoons granola
- 1 tablespoon honey (optional)

Instructions:

1. In a glass or bowl, layer Greek yogurt, blended berries, and granola.
2. If desired, drizzle with honey.
3. Partake in this healthy and fulfilling parfait!

Veggie Sticks with Hummus

Description:

Veggie Sticks and Hummus are the ideal combination of crunchy and creamy to up your snacking game. Loaded with nutrients and fiber, this tidbit keeps you empowered and fulfilled over the course of the day.

Serving Size: 1

Prep Time: 10 minutes

Cooking Time: 0 minutes

Ingredients:

- 1 cup baby carrots
- 1 cup cucumber, sliced
- 1 cup bell peppers, sliced
- 1/2 cup hummus

Instructions:

1. Orchestrate child carrots, cucumber cuts, and ringer pepper strips on a plate.
2. Present with hummus for plunging.
3. Partake in this reviving and supplement pressed nibble!

Almond Butter Banana Bites

Description:

Experience the ideal harmony between pleasantness and mash with Almond Margarine Banana Chomps. These reduced down treats are scrumptious as well as give a mix of sound fats, protein, and normal sugars.

Serving Size: 2

Prep Time: 10 minutes

Cooking Time: 0 minutes

Ingredients:

- 1 banana, sliced
- 2 tablespoons almond butter
- 2 tablespoons unsweetened shredded coconut

Instructions:

1. Spread almond margarine on banana cuts.
2. Sprinkle with coconut flakes.

3. Partake in this scrumptious and fulfilling nibble!

Trail Mix with Nuts and Seeds

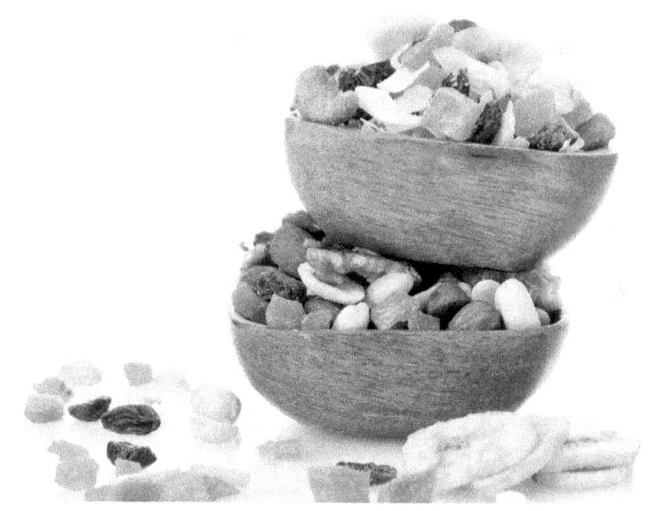

Description:

With nuts and seeds, you can make your own Trail Mix, which is a great snack for when you're on the go. Loaded with protein, fiber, and various surfaces, this blend keeps you energized and centered.

Serving Size: 1

Prep Time: 5 minutes

Cooking Time: 0 minutes

Ingredients:

- 1/4 cup almonds
- 1/4 cup walnuts
- 2 tablespoons pumpkin seeds
- 2 tablespoons dried cranberries
- 1 tablespoon dark chocolate chips

Instructions:

1. Mix almonds, walnuts, pumpkin seeds, dried cranberries, and dark chocolate chips in a bowl.
2. Portion into a snack-sized bag.
3. Enjoy this convenient and nutrient-dense trail mix!

Apple Slices with Peanut Butter

Description:

Fulfill your sweet and flavorful desires with Apple Cuts and Peanut Butter. This exemplary mix gives a mix of regular sugars, sound fats, and protein — a brilliant decision for a fast and scrumptious tidbit.

Serving Size: 1

Prep Time: 5 minutes

Cooking Time: 0 minutes

Ingredients:

- 1 apple, sliced
- 2 tablespoons peanut butter

Instructions:

1. Cut the apple into meager wedges.
2. Plunge each cut into peanut butter.
3. Partake in this scrumptious and nutritious tidbit!

Chia Seed Pudding with Berries

Description:

Experience a superb and supplement loaded nibble with Chia Seed Pudding and Berries. Wealthy in omega-3 unsaturated fats and cell reinforcements, this pudding is a brilliant decision for keeping up with energy levels.

Serving Size: 1

Prep Time: 5 minutes (plus chilling time)

Cooking Time: 0 minutes

Ingredients:

- 2 tablespoons chia seeds
- 1/2 cup almond milk
- 1/2 teaspoon vanilla extract
- 1/2 cup mixed berries (blueberries, raspberries)

Instructions:

1. In a container, blend chia seeds, almond milk, and vanilla concentrate.

2. Refrigerate for no less than 2 hours or short-term until it arrives at a pudding-like consistency.
3. Top with blended berries.
4. Take pleasure in this nutritious and delicious chia seed pudding!

Cottage Cheese and Pineapple Cups

Description:

Partake in a sweet and flavorful blend with Curds and Pineapple Cups. This healthy snack is a refreshing and satisfying option for smart snacking because it is loaded with vitamin C and protein.

Serving Size: 1

Prep Time: 5 minutes

Cooking Time: 0 minutes

Ingredients:

- 1/2 cup cottage cheese

- 1/2 cup pineapple chunks (fresh or canned)

Instructions:

1. Cottage cheese should fill a cup or bowl.

2. Top with pineapple pieces.

3. Partake in this basic and healthy tidbit!

Kale Chips with Parmesan

Description:

Kale Chips and Parmesan will satisfy your savory hankerings. Offering a boost of vitamins and minerals, this crunchy, flavorful snack is a smart alternative to conventional chips.

Serving Size: 1

Prep Time: 10 minutes

Cooking Time: 15 minutes

Ingredients:

- 2 cups kale, torn into bite-sized pieces

- 1 tablespoon olive oil

- 2 tablespoons grated Parmesan cheese
- Salt and pepper to taste

Instructions:

1. Preheat the broiler to 350°F (175°C).

2. Throw kale with olive oil, Parmesan cheddar, salt, and pepper.

3. Bake for 12 to 15 minutes, or until crispy, on a baking sheet.

4. Take pleasure in these tasty and guilt-free kale chips!

Edamame and Sea Salt Pods

Description:

Decide on a protein-stuffed and fulfilling nibble with Edamame and Ocean Salt Units. These steamed soybean units are heavenly as well as a helpful and careful decision for shrewd eating.

Serving Size: 1

Prep Time: 5 minutes

Cooking Time: 5 minutes

Ingredients:

- 1 cup edamame pods (frozen or fresh)
- Sea salt to taste

Instructions:

1. Edamame pods should be cooked in accordance with the package's instructions.
2. Sprinkle with ocean salt.
3. Enjoy this easy and healthy snack made with edamame!

Roasted Chickpeas with Smoky Paprika

Description:

Fulfill your flavorful desires with Cooked Chickpeas highlighting a smoky paprika contort. Loaded with protein and fiber, these crunchy nibbles are a tasty and brilliant option in contrast to customary tidbits.

Serving Size: 1

Prep Time: 10 minutes

Cooking Time: 40 minutes

Ingredients:

- 1 can chickpeas, drained and rinsed
- 1 tablespoon olive oil
- 1 teaspoon smoky paprika
- 1/2 teaspoon garlic powder
- 1/2 teaspoon cumin
- Salt to taste

Instructions:

1. Preheat the stove to 400°F (200°C) and line a baking sheet with material paper.
2. Wipe chickpeas off and throw with olive oil, smoky paprika, garlic powder, cumin, and salt.
3. On the baking sheet, arrange the chickpeas in a single layer.
4. Cook for 40 minutes or until brilliant and firm, shaking the dish infrequently.

5. Permit to cool prior to nibbling. Take pleasure in these savory and filling roasted chickpeas!

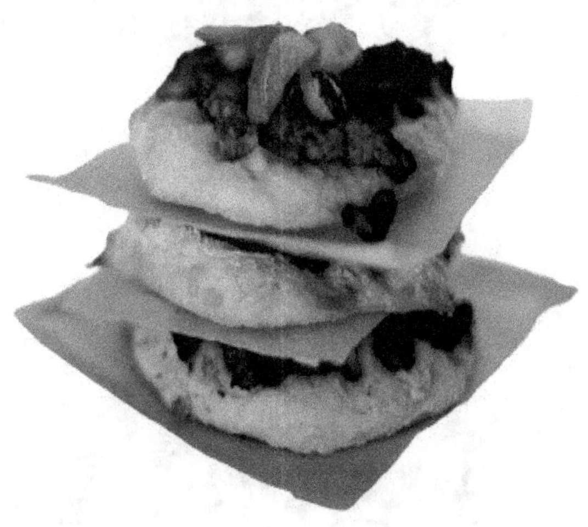

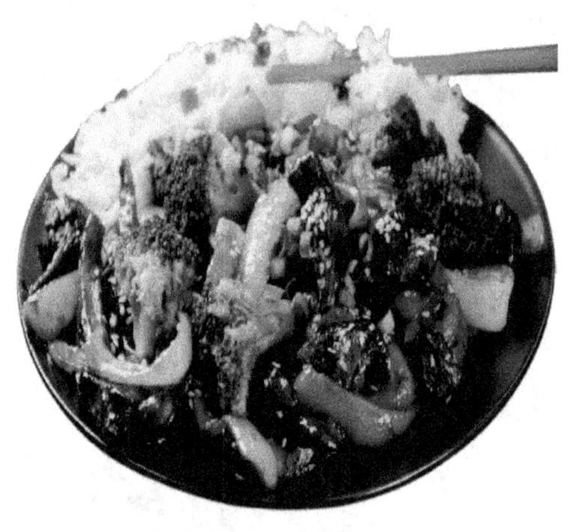

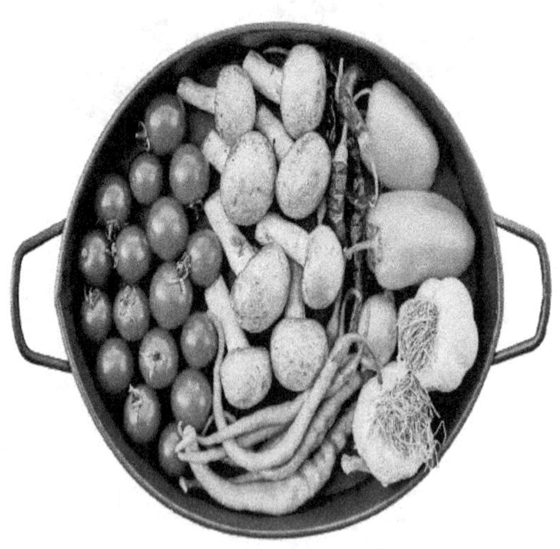

CHAPTER 7: SWEET TREATS WITH A PURPOSE

Healthy Banana Oat Muffins

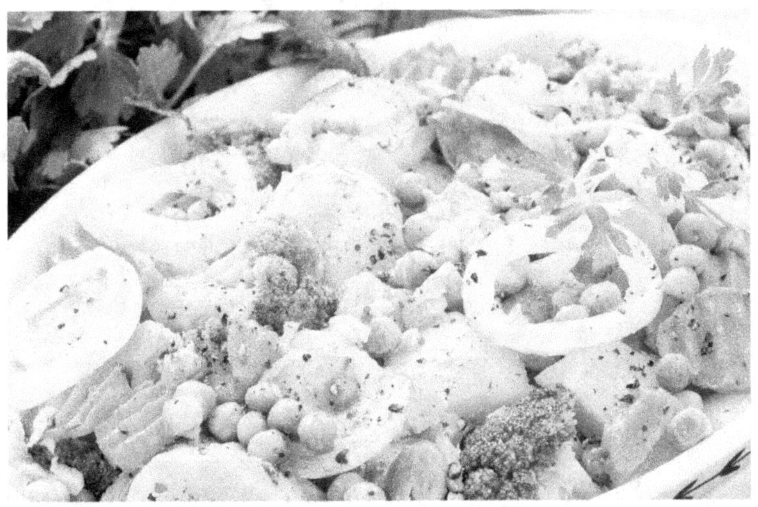

Description:

Enjoy virtuous pleasantness with Sound Banana Oat Biscuits. These clammy and tasty treats are normally improved with ready bananas and made with healthy fixings, giving a wonderful option in contrast to conventional biscuits.

Serving Size: 12

Prep Time: 15 minutes

Cooking Time: 20 minutes

Ingredients:

- 2 ripe bananas, mashed
- 1/2 cup unsweetened applesauce
- 1/4 cup honey or maple syrup
- 1/4 cup coconut oil, melted
- 1 teaspoon vanilla extract
- 2 cups rolled oats
- 1 teaspoon baking powder
- 1/2 teaspoon baking soda
- 1/2 teaspoon cinnamon
- Pinch of salt

Optional:

- chopped nuts or dark chocolate chips

Instructions:

1. Preheat the broiler to 350°F (175°C) and line a biscuit tin with liners.

2. In a bowl, blend pounded bananas, fruit purée, honey or maple syrup, softened coconut oil, and vanilla concentrate.

3. Add moved oats, baking powder, baking pop, cinnamon, and a spot of salt. Mix until all around joined.

4. Whenever wanted, overlay in hacked nuts or dull chocolate chips.

5. Split the hitter between the biscuit cups and heat for 20 minutes or until a toothpick tells the truth.

6. Take pleasure in these healthy banana oat muffins!

Avocado Chocolate Mousse

Description:

Experience the debauchery of chocolate mousse with a solid contort. Avocado Chocolate Mousse is a velvety and rich treat that involves avocados for a sleek surface and regular pleasantness.

Serving Size: 4

Prep Time: 10 minutes

Cooking Time: 0 minutes

Ingredients:

- 2 ripe avocados
- 1/4 cup unsweetened cocoa powder
- 1/4 cup maple syrup or agave nectar
- 1 teaspoon vanilla extract
- Pinch of salt
- Optional toppings: berries or a dollop of Greek yogurt

Instructions:

1. Scoop the tissue of the avocados into a blender or food processor.
2. Vanilla extract, maple syrup or agave nectar, cocoa powder, and a pinch of salt should be added.

3. Mix until smooth and rich.

4. Before serving, chill for at least 30 minutes in the refrigerator.

5. Top with berries or a dab of Greek yogurt whenever wanted.

6. Partake in this tasty and righteous avocado chocolate mousse!

Chia Seed Berry Pudding

Description:

Fulfill your sweet desires with Chia Seed Berry Pudding — a brilliant and supplement stuffed dessert. Chia seeds add a pudding-like consistency while berries bring regular pleasantness and cell reinforcements.

Serving Size: 2

Prep Time: 5 minutes (plus chilling time)

Cooking Time: 0 minutes

Ingredients:

- 1/4 cup chia seeds

- 1 cup almond milk

- 1 tablespoon honey or maple syrup

- 1/2 teaspoon vanilla extract

- 1 cup mixed berries (strawberries, blueberries, raspberries)

Instructions:

1. In a bowl, blend chia seeds, almond milk, honey or maple syrup, and vanilla concentrate.

2. Put it in the refrigerator for at least two hours or overnight until it has the consistency of pudding.

3. Before serving, top with a variety of berries.

4. Partake in this healthy and normally improved chia seed berry pudding!

Baked Apples with Cinnamon

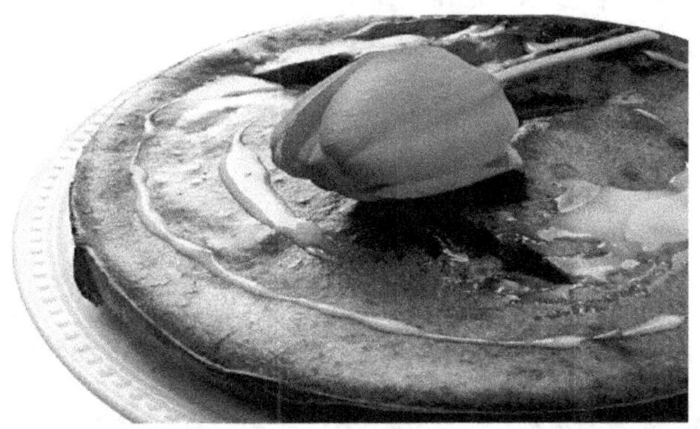

Description:

Experience the encouraging pleasantness of Prepared Apples with Cinnamon. This straightforward and nutritious sweet permits the regular sugars of apples to sparkle, with a dash of warm cinnamon for some extra zing.

Serving Size: 2

Prep Time: 10 minutes

Cooking Time: 30 minutes

Ingredients:

- 2 apples, cored and halved

- 1 tablespoon melted coconut oil

- 1 teaspoon cinnamon

- 1 tablespoon honey or maple syrup

- Optional: cleaved nuts or a sprinkle of almond spread

Instructions:

1. Preheat the broiler to 375°F (190°C) and line a baking dish with material paper.

2. Place apple parts in the dish.

3. In a bowl, blend dissolved coconut oil, cinnamon, and honey or maple syrup.

4. Bake for 30 minutes, or until the apples are tender, brushing the mixture over them.

5. **Optional:** Sprinkle with hacked nuts or shower with almond margarine prior to serving.

6. Partake in these warm and encouraging prepared apples!

Coconut and Berry Nice Cream

Description:

Coconut and Berry Nice Cream, a dairy-free and naturally sweetened alternative to traditional ice cream, is the perfect way to cool down. Mixing frozen berries with velvety coconut milk makes a delectable and irreproachable sweet.

Serving Size: 4

Prep Time: 5 minutes (plus freezing time)

Cooking Time: 0 minutes

Ingredients:

- 2 cups frozen mixed berries
- 1 can full-fat coconut milk, chilled
- 1/4 cup honey or maple syrup
- 1 teaspoon vanilla extract

Optional:

- toppings of fresh berries or shredded coconut

Instructions:

1. Blend the chilled coconut milk, vanilla extract, honey or maple syrup, and frozen berries in a blender.

2. Mix until smooth and velvety.

3. Scoop into bowls and top with destroyed coconut or new berries whenever wanted.

4. Freeze for an extra 1-2 hours for a firmer surface.

5. Enjoy this coconut and berry nice cream, which is both refreshing and purposeful!

Healthy Chicken and Vegetable Sheet Pan Dinner

Description:

Improve on your supper arrangement with this sound chicken and vegetable sheet container supper. Loaded with vivid veggies and lean protein, this one-dish wonder makes cleanup a breeze while giving a fair and supporting dinner.

Serving Size: 4

Prep Time: 15 minutes

Cooking Time: 25 minutes

Ingredients:

- 4 boneless, skinless chicken breasts
- 1 pound baby potatoes, halved
- 1 cup baby carrots
- 1 cup broccoli florets
- 1 cup cherry tomatoes, halved
- 2 tablespoons olive oil
- 1 teaspoon garlic powder
- 1 teaspoon onion powder
- 1 teaspoon dried thyme
- Salt and pepper to taste
- Fresh parsley for garnish

Instructions:

1. Preheat the stove to 425°F (220°C) and line a baking sheet with material paper.

2. Place chicken bosoms, child potatoes, child carrots, broccoli, and cherry tomatoes on the sheet.

3. Shower with olive oil and sprinkle with garlic powder, onion powder, dried thyme, salt, and pepper.

4. Spread into a single layer after tossing to evenly coat everything.

5. Heat for 25 minutes or until the chicken is cooked through.

6. Decorate with new parsley and serve.

Stuffed Bell Peppers with Ground Turkey and Quinoa

Description:

Experience a generous and healthy supper with these stuffed chime peppers loaded up with a delightful combination of ground turkey and quinoa. This family-accommodating dish is both encouraging and nutritious, making it an ideal expansion to your supper turn.

Serving Size: 4

Prep Time: 20 minutes

Cooking Time: 40 minutes

Ingredients:

- 4 bell peppers, halved and seeds removed
- 1 cup quinoa, cooked
- 1 pound ground turkey
- 1 onion, finely chopped
- 2 cloves garlic, minced
- 1 can black beans, drained and rinsed
- 1 cup corn kernels
- 1 cup tomato sauce
- 1 teaspoon cumin

- 1 teaspoon chili powder
- Salt and pepper to taste
- Shredded cheddar cheese for topping
- Fresh cilantro for garnish

Instructions:

1. Preheat the stove to 375°F (190°C) and oil a baking dish.
2. In a skillet, cook ground turkey, onions, and garlic until the turkey is seared.
3. Add cooked quinoa, dark beans, corn, pureed tomatoes, cumin, stew powder, salt, and pepper. Stew for 10 minutes.
4. Fill each ringer pepper half with the turkey and quinoa blend.
5. Top with destroyed cheddar and prepare for 30 minutes or until peppers are delicate.
6. Embellish with new cilantro and serve.

Mushroom and Spinach Stuffed Chicken Breast

Description:

Raise your supper with these mushroom and spinach stuffed chicken bosoms. The blend of exquisite mushrooms, delicate spinach, and succulent chicken makes a tasty and outwardly engaging dish that is ideally suited for an extraordinary night feast.

Serving Size: 2

Prep Time: 15 minutes

Cooking Time: 30 minutes

Ingredients:

- 2 boneless, skinless chicken breasts
- 1 cup mushrooms, finely chopped
- 2 cups fresh spinach, chopped
- 1/2 cup feta cheese, crumbled
- 2 cloves garlic, minced
- 2 tablespoons olive oil

- Salt and pepper to taste

- Paprika for garnish

- Fresh parsley for garnish

Instructions:

1. Preheat the broiler to 375°F (190°C).

2. In a container, sauté mushrooms and garlic in olive oil until mellowed.

3. Add cleaved spinach and cook until withered.

4. Eliminate from intensity and mix in feta cheddar.

5. Cut a pocket into every chicken bosom and stuff with the mushroom and spinach blend.

6. Season the beyond the chicken bosoms with salt, pepper, and paprika.

7. Heat for 25-30 minutes or until the chicken is cooked through.

8. Decorate with new parsley and serve.

Quinoa and Black Bean Stuffed Acorn Squash

Description:

With these quinoa and black bean stuffed acorn squash, you can enjoy the flavors of fall. This dinner option is a hearty and satisfying choice for a cozy evening meal and is packed with a nutritious combination of quinoa, black beans, and autumn spices.

Serving Size: 4

Prep Time: 20 minutes

Cooking Time: 40 minutes

Ingredients:

- 2 acorn squash, halved and seeds removed
- 1 cup quinoa, cooked
- 1 can black beans, drained and rinsed
- 1/2 cup red onion, finely chopped
- 1/2 cup corn kernels

- 1 teaspoon cumin
- 1/2 teaspoon cinnamon
- Salt and pepper to taste
- 1/4 cup feta cheese, crumbled
- Fresh cilantro for garnish

Instructions:

- Preheat the broiler to 375°F (190°C) and line a baking sheet with material paper.
- Put oak seed squash parts on the sheet, cut side down, and heat for 20 minutes.
- In a bowl, blend cooked quinoa, dark beans, red onion, corn, cumin, cinnamon, salt, and pepper.
- Flip the squash parts, stuff with the quinoa blend, and prepare for 20 extra minutes.
- Embellish with disintegrated feta cheddar and new cilantro.
- Serve and partake in this great and sustaining supper!

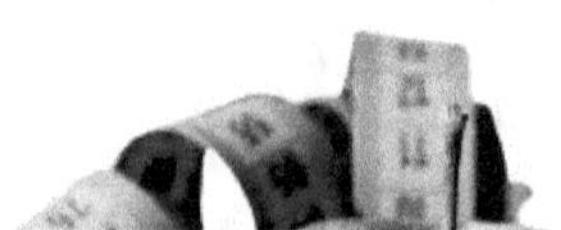

Chapter 8: Dining Out on the Glucose Revolution

Welcome to the interesting excursion of eating out while embracing the Glucose Unrest! This section fills in as your complete manual for exploring café menus with certainty, settling on glucose-accommodating decisions, and flawlessly integrating the standards of this progressive methodology into get-togethers and festivities.

Feast with Certainty: Exploring Café Menus

Leaving on the Glucose Insurgency doesn't mean saying goodbye to the delight of eating out. All things considered, it enables you to go with educated and pleasant decisions. Get familiar with the specialty of filtering menus with an insightful eye, recognizing choices that line up with glucose-accommodating standards without forfeiting flavor.

Key Issues:

Decoding the menu: Ace the expertise of unraveling menu depictions, perceiving stowed away sugars, and understanding the effect of different cooking strategies on the glycemic list.

Savvy Replacements: Learn how to adapt dishes to meet your glucose requirements more effectively. From trading refined sugars for entire grains to selecting lean protein sources, get familiar with the craft of making shrewd replacements without compromising taste.

Ways to settle on Glucose-Accommodating Decisions

Eating out ought not be a wellspring of stress; it ought to be a superb encounter. This part outfits you with down to earth ways to settle on glucose-accommodating decisions, guaranteeing that your eating experience adjusts flawlessly with your wellbeing objectives.

Key Points:

Adjusted Plates: Investigate the idea of making adjusted plates that consolidate lean proteins, sound fats, and complex carbs in amicable extents to help stable blood glucose levels.

Segment Control: Reveal procedures for overseeing segment sizes at eateries, forestalling overindulgence while as yet enjoying the kinds of your number one dishes.

Hydration Propensities: Find out why it's so important to stay hydrated while you eat and which beverages are good for you because of their low glucose content to pair with your meal.

Techniques for Get-togethers and Festivities

Get-togethers and festivities are a vital piece of life, and the Glucose Upheaval urges you to explore these events with elegance and care. This section gives you great ways to stay on track with your glucose goals while having fun with other people.

Key Themes:

Pre-Occasion Arrangement: Furnish yourself with pre-occasion systems, from eating a reasonable feast in advance to conveying your dietary inclinations to occasion coordinators. These means guarantee that you're gotten in a good position.

Making Conscious Decisions at Events: Investigate ways of going with glucose-accommodating decisions in assorted group environments, from mixed drink gatherings to family festivities. Find how to relish the experience without undermining your wellbeing objectives.

Indulgences for the Holidays: Discover how to celebrate special occasions without feeling guilty. Figure out how to appreciate treats with some restraint and relish the celebrations while holding your glucose levels in line.

End

Eating out isn't just about sustaining your body yet additionally about interfacing with others and enjoying valuable's experiences. The Glucose Upset enables you to easily accomplish this equilibrium. Embrace the information and methodologies introduced in this section, permitting you to eat out with certainty, settle on glucose-accommodating decisions, and happily partake in get-togethers and festivities. Allow the Glucose Revolution to enhance your dining experiences as well as your health!

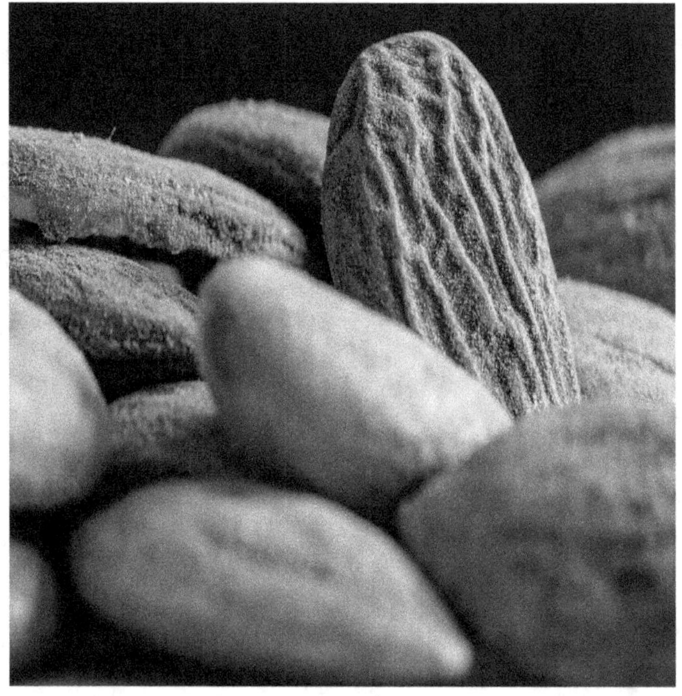

Chapter 9: Incorporating Physical Activity

Welcome to a crucial section of the Glucose Revolution, where we investigate the dynamic synergy between glucose management and physical activity. Discover fitness routines that align with the Glucose Revolution's principles and seamlessly incorporate movement into your daily life with the help of this chapter, which serves as your gateway to understanding the profound effect that exercise has on glucose levels.

The Job of Practice in Glucose The executives

Open the extraordinary force of actual work chasing ideal glucose the executives. This segment digs into the science behind what exercise means for blood glucose levels, offering bits of knowledge that enable you to pursue informed choices for your wellbeing.

Key Subjects:

Glucose Guideline: Figure out the unpredictable connection between actual work and glucose guideline, acquiring a complete comprehension of what exercise means for insulin responsiveness and glucose usage.

Effects Following Exercise: Examine the positive effects that exercise has on glucose levels afterward, such as an extended period of enhanced glucose uptake and improved insulin sensitivity, which have a positive ripple effect on overall metabolic health.

Wellness Schedules That Supplement the Glucose Upset

Find a variety of wellness schedules custom fitted to supplement the standards of the Glucose Transformation. Whether you're a carefully prepared wellness devotee or simply leaving on your excursion, these schedules offer assortment and viability in advancing glucose-accommodating activity.

Key Points:

Cardiovascular Activities: Embrace cardiovascular exercises like energetic strolling, cycling, and swimming, upgrading your heart wellbeing while at the same time supporting glucose guideline.

Strength Preparing: Uncover the advantages of integrating strength preparing into your daily practice. From further developing bulk to improving insulin awareness, strength preparing turns into an indispensable part of your glucose-accommodating wellness venture.

Connection Between the Mind and the Body: Investigate the significant effect of psyche body practices like yoga and jujitsu on pressure decrease and mental prosperity — basic components in keeping up with stable glucose levels.

Coordinating Development Into Day to day existence

This part reclassifies the idea of activity by underscoring the significance of reliable development all through your day to day routine. Figure out how little, deliberate activities can collect to make an underpinning of dynamic living.

Key Issues:

Deskercise Methods: Investigate work area well disposed practices intended to check the stationary impacts of office work. Learn how to inject vitality into your workday through discrete strength-building exercises and stretches.

Dynamic Transportation: Embrace dynamic transportation strategies, like strolling or cycling, to consistently coordinate active work into your everyday drive. Upgrade your prosperity while diminishing your carbon impression.

Practical Wellness: Submerge yourself in the idea of utilitarian wellness, stressing developments that improve your capacity to perform ordinary exercises. This approach guarantees that exercise is certainly not a different substance however a basic piece of your life.

Conclusion At the end of this chapter, you are ready to use the transformative power of physical activity in your journey toward glucose management. You are at the intersection of knowledge and action. Embrace the standards, take on the different wellness schedules, and mesh development consistently into your everyday existence. The mix of activity into the Glucose Upset isn't just about wellness; it's a comprehensive obligation to your wellbeing, guaranteeing that each step, stretch, or breath adds to the essentialness and equilibrium you look for. Leave the excursion to ideal glucose the board alone as animating as the proactive tasks that impel you forward. Welcome to a daily existence where development isn't simply a decision yet a festival of your prosperity.

CONCLUSION:

Additional Resources

Embracing a Lively Way of life with the Glucose Insurgency Diet Cookbook

As we bid goodbye to the Glucose Unrest Diet Cookbook, we consider the extraordinary excursion it has cleared for innumerable people looking for an amicable connection between nourishment, prosperity, and the delight of living. This cookbook isn't only an assortment of recipes; It serves as a guide, a friend, and a springboard for a life filled with purpose.

Celebrating Creative Cuisine:

The Glucose Insurgency Diet Cookbook welcomes you to commend the imaginativeness of culinary innovativeness. Every recipe is a demonstration of the thought that feeding the body need not be a penance but rather a magnificent investigation. From invigorating morning meals to supporting meals, the cookbook offers an orchestra of flavors that make each dinner a festival of prosperity.

Engaging Through Information:

Past the kitchen, the Glucose Upheaval Diet Cookbook engages with information. It demystifies the many-sided connection between diet, blood glucose levels, and in general wellbeing. It inspires a lifestyle rooted in balance and vitality by providing you with the knowledge necessary to make informed decisions through informative chapters.

All encompassing Way of life Change:

This cookbook is certainly not a transitory fix; it's an impetus for an all encompassing way of life change. It interlaces the standards of careful eating, actual work, and a positive outlook. It's a challenge to embrace the Glucose Unrest not as an inflexible arrangement of rules but rather as an adaptable and manageable way to deal with prosperity.

A People group of Help:
The Glucose Unrest Diet Cookbook stretches out past its pages, cultivating a local area of help. From online discussions to selective online classes, it makes spaces for shared encounters, consolation, and aggregate development. The journey toward optimal health becomes a shared and uplifting experience in this community, where people find strength in unity.

Supporting Energetic Wellbeing:
As you close the cookbook, convey the soul of the Glucose Unrest into your regular routine. Allow it to be a directing light towards supported dynamic wellbeing, an update that each decision matters, and

that prosperity is an excursion, not an objective. Wishing you many more culinary adventures, mindful movement, and a profound sense of vitality in the years to come.